Cop\

MW01489850

Contents

What is a low-fiber (low-residue) diet?

A low-residue diet is a diet that is designed to "rest" the bowel. It is a type of low-fiber diet with added restrictions. A low-residue diet is not a diet plan to follow regularly. It is advised for some people for the short term during a flare of inflammatory bowel disease here is intestinal narrowing, before or after bowel surgery, and other conditions for which it is useful to reduce the amount of stool in the intestines.

The food we eat is digested so that the body can extract the nutrients it needs to function. What's left over is "residue" or undigested food that passes through the colon (large intestine), and is eliminated as stool or feces. A low-residue diet limits fiber and other substances with the goal of reducing stool volume. This results in fewer and smaller bowel movements, potentially relieving symptoms of bowel diseases that can cause inflammation, such as abdominal pain and cramping, bloating, and gas formation.

Who is a low-fiber diet plan for?

In disease and conditions in which the colon has the potential to be inflamed, a low-fiber diet may "rest" the colon. The low-residue diet limits the amount of work the colon has to do in forming feces because most of the content of the diet is absorbed and less waste is required to be eliminated. Since there is a reduced quantity of stool, the time it takes to pass through the length of the colon is increased, resulting in smaller, less frequent bowel movements.

Low-fiber diets are often recommended for patients with a number of different conditions, including the following:

• Flares of inflammatory bowel disease, either Crohn's Disease or ulcerative colitis

• Vowel tumors

• Inflamed bowel due to radiation or chemotherapy treatments

• Before or after bowel surgery, or before colonoscopy

• Inflammation or narrowing of the bowel

In the past, individuals with diverticulosis or irritable bowel disease syndrome (IBS) might have been prescribed a low-residue diet; however, current recommendations now suggest that a high fiber diet might be of more benefit in these conditions. Special diets may be prescribed during flares of acute bowel inflammation (as with diverticulitis), but a high-fiber diet is generally recommended for people with the diverticular disease as this has been shown to be protective for the development of diverticula.

Any diet like this one that restricts certain foods may also be responsible for the decreased intake of important minerals and vitamins. Calcium, potassium, folic acid, and vitamin C supplements may be required with a low-fiber diet.

Individuals on a low-fiber diet will want to limit their fiber intake to 7-10 grams per day. Read food labels carefully. Most food packaging will list the amount of fiber on their label.

What can you eat on a low fiber diet?

Typically, a low fiber diet limits fiber intake to around 10 grams per dayTrusted Source for both males and females. It also reduces other foods that might stimulate bowel activity.

The foods that make up the low fiber diet are not the best options for long-term health.

For instance, whole grain bread has more nutrients and health benefits than white bread, but whole-grains are high in fiber, so people on this diet should opt for white bread instead.

Your doctor will recommend that you only follow the low fiber diet for a short time — until your bowel heals, diarrhea resolves, or your body has recovered from surgery.

Foods to eat

Proper nutrition is crucial for the best management of IBD and other conditions that affect the bowel.

Some people only follow a low-fiber diet for short periods, while others may use it as a long-term strategy. Even if just following the diet for a for a short time, it is still important to try and eat a variety of foods.

The following foods may be included as part of a low-fiber diet, depending on individual symptoms and tolerance:

Low fiber foods

- white bread, white pasta, and white rice

- foods made with refined white flour, such as pancakes and bagels

- low fiber cereal, hot or cold

- canned vegetables

- fresh vegetables, in small amounts, if they are well-cooked

- potatoes without the skin

- eggs

- dairy products, if your body can process them well

- tender protein sources, such as eggs, tofu, chicken, and fish

- creamy peanut butter

- fats, including olive oil, mayonnaise, gravy, and butter

Low fiber fruits

- fruit juices without pulp

- canned fruit

- cantaloupe

- honeydew melon

- watermelon

- nectarines

- papayas

- peaches

- plums

Low fiber vegetables

- well-cooked or canned vegetables without seeds or skins

- carrots

- beets

- asparagus tips

- white potatoes without skin

- string beans

- lettuce, if your body can tolerate it

- tomato sauces

- acorn squash without seeds

- pureed spinach

- strained vegetable juice

- cucumbers without seeds or skin, zucchini, and shredded lettuce are fine to eat raw

Avoid any food that you know your body will find it difficult to digest.

When you're going on a low fiber diet, certain foods — like spicy foods — may affect your digestive system more. You might also want to avoid tea, coffee, and alcohol during this time.

Foods to avoid

Foods to avoid on a low-fiber diet:

- Breakfast cereals, including muesli, bran flakes, puffed wheat, shredded wheat, porridge, granola, or cereals with added dried fruits.

- Whole-wheat bread, seeded loaves, and bread with added fruit, nuts, or seeds.

- All vegetable skins, peels, and seeds, including potato skins.

- Whole-wheat or brown pasta or grains, including brown or wild rice, bulgar wheat, quinoa, and couscous.

- Cakes or pastries with nuts, fruits, or seeds, including fig rolls, flapjacks, and fruit scones.

- Fruits with seeds and peels still attached, including raspberries, strawberries, blueberries, blackcurrants, passion fruit, kiwi, oranges, coconut, and fresh figs.

- All dried fruit, such as figs, prunes, dates, and raisins.

- Any raw, uncooked vegetables.

- Pulses, such as lentils, baked beans, kidney beans, and chickpeas.

- Seeds, such as pumpkin, sunflower, and flaxseeds.

Meal plan

Meal options for someone following the low-fiber diet include:

Breakfast:

- low-fiber cereal (for example Rice Krispies, Cornflakes, Special K) with milk or non-dairy milk

- white bread or toast with butter and jelly

- poached eggs

Mid-morning snack:

- crumpet

- smooth yogurt or kefir

- applesauce with cinnamon

Lunch:

- a sandwich made from white bread with slices of turkey breast

- white pasta with tuna

Mid-afternoon snack:

- ripe banana

- plain biscuits

- pudding

- canned mandarin oranges

Dinner:

- white rice with salmon and low-fiber vegetables

- omelet

- chicken breast with mashed potato

Tips

When introducing new foods, add only one at a time. This will help a person identify foods that make their symptoms worse.

Read the labels on pre-prepared or packaged meals, as they may contain ingredients that trigger symptoms.

Avoid anything with bits in it, including yogurts, marmalade, mustard, popcorn, and crunchy peanut butter.

Here are some more useful tips for a low-fiber diet:

- sieve soups and lumpy stews

- eat small meals every 3–4 hours

- chew food slowly and thoroughly

- avoid large quantities of caffeine or alcohol

- avoid rich sauces and spicy foods

- consume only small amounts of dairy

- avoid fizzy drinks

- speak to a dietitian about what fruits and vegetables are safe to eat

Recovery

If eating or digestion continues to be difficult or painful, it is essential to speak to a doctor. People with IBD may need considerable support from a dietitian to manage the disease during times of relapse and remission.

While much research is conflicting on the best dietary approach to prevent or delay IBD relapse, there is some evidenceTrusted Source that supports a semi-vegetarian diet and exclusion diets.

It is vital to eat a varied diet that contains all of the essential nutrients and enough calories to maintain energy levels.

Why is a low fiber diet beneficial?

A low fiber diet can help give your digestive system a break. Fiber, while it usually has health benefits, takes more effort for your body to digest.

Your doctor might recommend trying this diet for a short time if you have one of the following:

- IBS

- Crohn's disease

- ulcerative colitis

- diverticulitis

- diarrhea

- abdominal cramps

- constipation

- irritation or damage in the digestive tract

- bowel narrowing caused by a tumor

- recovery from gastrointestinal surgery, including colostomy and ileostomy

- current radiation therapy or other treatments that might affect the gastrointestinal tract

How to start eating fiber again

When you're ready to start introducing fiber again, it's best to do this slowly. This is help prevent uncomfortable side effects.

Increase intake gradually by 5 grams of fiber per week. To do this, try introducing a small portion of one high fiber food per day.

If the food doesn't cause symptoms, you can add it back into your diet.

How much fiber you need is based on your age and sex. According to the Academy of Nutrition and Dietetics, people following a 2,000-calorie diet should get the following amounts of fiber:

- 38 grams per day for adult males, and 30 grams after age 50

- 25 grams per day for adult females, and 21 grams after age 50

The most healthful way to get fiber is by eating fruits with skins left on, vegetables, whole grains, beans, nuts, and seeds.

Know your fibers

There are two types of fiber:

• Soluble fiber. This type of fiber absorbs water during digestion, turning into a soft, gel-like substance. For some, soluble fiber is less likely to irritate the digestive tract. Others may notice an increase in gas, bloating, or discomfort since many soluble fiber-rich foods also contain fermentable fibers or prebiotics that feed gut bacteria. Still, during a low fiber diet, small amounts of soluble fiber might be okay. Beans, oats, peas, and citrus fruits are high in soluble fiber.

• Insoluble fiber. This type of fiber does not dissolve in the stomach, and the undigested fragments may irritate the gut. During a low fiber diet, be especially careful to avoid foods like whole wheat, grains, and fruit and veggie skins.

LOW FIBER DIET RECIPES

Trying new low fiber-friendly recipes is a great way to explore new flavors and find new favorite dishes while looking after your health. In this part are nourishing low fiber diet recipes for you to enjoy and ease your digestion.

Tasty Three-Fish Terrine

Preparation time

50 minutes

Ingredients:

- 3 1/2 ounces salmon fillet

- 7 ounces fresh haddock fillet

- 3 1/2 ounces undyed smoked haddock fillet

- 3 1/2 fluid ounces heavy cream

- 2 large eggs, beaten

- Salt and pepper

- Paprika

- 1 teaspoon lemon juice and lemon wedges

- Large handful of mache

Instructions:

1. Preheat oven to 400° F.

2. Oil four ramekins and sprinkle with paprika.

3. Cut the salmon fillet into thin strips and divide between the ramekins, laying them neatly.

4. Blend the smoked fish in a food processor, add 1/3 of the beaten egg mixture and 1/3 of the cream, blending until smooth. Set aside.

5. Blend together the fresh haddock and the remaining eggs and cream, adding a pinch of salt and pepper, a teaspoon of lemon juice and a pinch of paprika.

6. Place a tablespoon of the smoked fish mixture in each ramekin and top with fresh haddock mixture.

7. Press lightly to smooth.

8. Place the ramekins into a roasting tray; pour some boiling water into the tray so that it comes up about 2/3 of the way.

9. Bake in the oven for 30 minutes.

10. Turn upside down on a plate and garnish with mache and a lemon wedge to serve!

Simple Chicken-Veggie Pasta Soup

Preparation time

15 minutes

Ingredients:

- 2 cans (14 ounces) pear halves or quarters in juice

- 1 cup self-raising flour

- 2 tablespoons cocoa powder

- 1/2 cup fine sugar

- 2/3 cup butter, plus extra for dish

- 2 medium eggs

- 2 teaspoons vanilla extract

Instructions:

1. Place broth, carrot and potato in a small saucepan.

2. Bring to a boil, then reduce heat and cook until vegetables are tender.

3. Add tomatoes and asparagus tips and cook until asparagus is tender.

4. Stir in cooked pasta and cook until heated through.

Beautifully Basic Beef Tacos

Preparation time

12 minutes

Ingredients:

- 6 corn taco shells

- 1/2 pound lean ground beef

- 1 tablespoon canola oil

- 1 cup onion, chopped

- 1 clove garlic, minced

- 1 teaspoon chili powder

- 1/2 teaspoon black pepper

- 1/4 teaspoon ground cumin

- 1/4 teaspoon hot sauce

- 3/4 cup shredded lettuce

- 6 tablespoons chopped tomato

- 6 tablespoons shredded sharp cheddar cheese

Instructions:

1. Brown the ground beef over medium heat in a large frying pan.

2. Drain well, remove from the pan and set aside.

3. Heat the oil in the pan and add 1/2 cup of chopped onion.

4. Cook until clear.

5. Add garlic. Cook and stir for one minute.

6. Add cooked beef back into the pan.

7. Stir in chili powder, pepper, cumin and hot sauce.

8. Remove from heat.

9. Add 1/4 cup of the meat mixture inside each taco shell.

10. Top with 2 tablespoons of lettuce, 1 tablespoon each of tomato, cheese and remaining onion.

Savory Beet Carrot Soup

Preparation time

15 minutes

Ingredients:

- 4 cups vegetable broth

- 1 carrot, sliced

- 1 can beets, cooked

- salt to taste

- nonfat yogurt for serving (if desired)

Instructions:

1. Place sliced carrot and vegetable broth in a small saucepan.

2. Bring to a boil, then reduce heat and cook covered until carrots are tender.

3. Add beets and cook until heated through

4. Pour soup into a blender and puree until smooth.

5. Season to taste with salt.

6. Serve with a dollop of yogurt stirred in if desired.

Pear and Cocoa Pudding

Preparation time

40 minutes

Ingredients:

- 2 cans (14 ounces) pear halves or quarters in juice

- 1 cup self-raising flour

- 2 tablespoons cocoa powder

- 1/2 cup fine sugar

- 2/3 cup butter, plus extra for dish

- 2 medium eggs

- 2 teaspoons vanilla extract

Instructions

1. Preheat oven to 400° F.

2. Drain the pears and lay in a pie dish or other ovenproof dish.

3. Add remaining ingredients to a food processor and blend until completely smooth.

4. Drop spoonfuls of batter over the pears and carefully spread with a wet spoon.

5. Bake for 25-30 minutes.

6. Allow to cool for a few minutes before serving.

Eggy Devils

Preparation time

20 minutes

Ingredients

- 3 tablespoons whole egg organic mayonnaise

- 6 free range eggs

- Pinch of turmeric powder

- Pinch of mustard powder

- Salt and pepper to taste

- Paprika to dust eggs with

- Packet of water crackers

Instructions

1. Add eggs to a saucepan, cover with water and heat.

2. Once boiling, let the eggs cook for 4 ½ minutes.

3. Remove from heat and place the eggs into cold water for one minute then carefully peel and slice them in half lengthwise.

4. Gently scoop out the yolks into a bowl and mash with the mayonnaise, turmeric, mustard and salt and pepper to taste.

5. Cut a little slice off the rounded bottom of the egg white halves so they sit firmly on the plate or cracker without wobbling, then pipe or spoon the yolk mix back into the white egg halves.

6. Dust the tops lightly with paprika and serve.

Lemongrass Beef

Preparation time

20 minutes

Ingredients

- 2 tablespoons sesame oil

- 1 tablespoon fish sauce

- 2 tablespoons sweet chili sauce

- 2 packets microwave basmati rice

- 2 teaspoons shredded coconut

- 1 tablespoon lemongrass paste

- 500 grams lean grass-fed beef mince

- 1 tube or tub Gourmet Thai seasoning stir in paste

- 100 grams of peeled Lebanese cucumber cut into chunks

- 2 carrots peeled and julienned

- 50 grams salted peanuts

- 1/4 cup chopped thai basil (for decorating)

- 1 lime cut into 4 to serve.

Instructions

1. Heat a wok and add thai seasoning, fish sauce and lemongrass paste and sesame oil, stir quickly and then add the minced beef

2. Stir for 3-4 minutes until browned

3. Cook the ready to each rice packet as per instructions and when ready add a teaspoon of shredded coconut to each packet and stir through being careful not to burn yourself with the hot steam.

4. Dived the mince, rice, cucumber, carrots in a bowl and sprinkle the Thai basil evenly on top and add a dash of sweet chilli sauce and serve with lime quarter

Pulled Chicken Salad

Preparation time

25 minutes

Ingredients

- 200 grams cooked pulled BBQ chicken

- 1/3 cup drained tinned apricots thinly sliced

- 100 grams dry weight of orzo pasta

- 150 grams baby spinach with stalks removed

- 70 grams fontina cheese (or cheddar) cut into small cubes

- 30 grams parmesan cheese

- 1/4 cup finely chopped parsley

- 1/3 cup Chang's ® fried noodles

- 5 tablespoon olive oil

- 3 tablespoon red wine vinegar

- salt and pepper to taste

Instructions

1. Shred cooked cooled chicken with a fork

2. Place cooked cooled orzo pasta in a microwave dish mix through fontina and parmesan cheese and microwave for 1-2 minutes until cheese has just melted, mix through the pasta

3. Let the bowl cool add spinach, parsley, chicken, and apricots and blend evenly through the salad

4. Mix olive oil and red wine vinegar with salt and pepper blend well and pour on the salad. Mix through

5. Add the crispy noodles just before serving to maintain their crunch

6. Serve on its own or with crusty white Ciabatta and olive oil dip.

Turkish Bake

Preparation time

1 hour 20 minutes

Ingredients

- 250 grams grated zucchini (let the zucchini settle on paper towels to drain excess moisture for 10 minutes, squeeze it a little more to get out the rest of the moisture and then use it)

- 1/4 cup chives (finely chopped)

- 1/2 teaspoon garlic powder

- 1/4 cup fresh dill (chopped)

- 1 teaspoon coriander powder

- 1 teaspoon baking powder

- 60 grams white flour

- 120 grams feta cheese crumbled (or vegan feta)

- 3 eggs or ORGRAN ® vegan easy egg made to specification

- 25 ml extra virgin olive oil

- salt and pepper to taste

Instructions

1. Preheat the oven to 180C fan forced

2. Grease and line a baking loaf tin with baking paper. In a large bowl mix the chives, zucchini, baking powder, flour, crumbled feta, olive oil, coriander powder, dill herb, and garlic powder and mix thoroughly.

3. Whisk eggs (or egg substitute) and combine evenly with the mixture.

4. Place in the loaf tin and bake for 30 minutes.

5. Remove from oven to check if there is still some moisture in the middle of the loaf by pressing down on the loaf.

6. Return to oven for a further 23-27 minutes or until the mixture is set.

7. Let the loaf stand in the pan for 10 minutes before serving.

8. Serve with lemon wedges, extra dill and mint, Turkish bread and yogurt if desired.

Pho Delicious

Preparation time

25 minutes

Ingredients

- 1000 ml Vietnamese inspired chicken Pho liquid

- 1250 grams skinless chicken thighs (cut into 2.5cm chunks)

- 500 grams (uncooked weight) rice noodles (cooked and ready to add to the soup)

- 5 tablespoons Extra virgin olive oil

- 1 1/4 cup chopped coriander

- 1 1/4 cup mint leaves

- 1 1/4 cup bean sprouts*

- 2 1/2 lime (quartered)

- 2 1/2 peeled julienned carrot

- salt and pepper to taste

Instructions

1. In a large heavy bottomed saucepan add the olive oil and heat to medium.

2. Add the chunks of chicken and cook until surfaces are brown

3. Let cool for a minute and add stock and bring to the boil then simmer until the chicken is cooked through approximately 15 minutes

4. Warm four bowls

5. Place the cooked noodles in the bowls, add bean sprouts, coriander and mint to each bowl and spoon in the hot soup adding chicken to each dish

6. Decorate with lime quarter

Apple Sausage Pasta

Preparation time

30 minutes

Ingredients

- 450 grams chicken sausages (or veggie sausages)

- 1 Green apple (peeled, cored and chopped into chunks)

- 1/2 large brown onion (finely diced)

- 2 tsp garlic powder

- 500 ml low salt chicken/vegetable stock

- 400 ml pasata

- 300 grams pasta

- 1 cup shredded cheddar cheese

- 1 tbsp extra-virgin olive oil

- salt and pepper to taste

Instructions

1. In a large frying pan (must have a lid) add the olive oil and heat to medium heat.

2. Cook the onions, garlic and sausages for about 10 minutes until golden.

3. Let the sausages cool and slice them thinly and add back to the pan and heat again to medium with the chopped apple until apple is soft.

4. Add the stock and pasata, stirring to ensure the mixture is blended through, add salt and pepper to taste and bring to a boil.

5. Add the pasta and the lid and cook until the pasta is cooked, stirring regularly to ensure the pasta does not stick at the bottom of the pan.

6. Stir until the liquid has evaporated, stir cheese through at the last minute.

7. Serve with a side of steamed vegetables.

Pink Lady Smoothie

Preparation time

15 minutes

Ingredients

- 350 ml water or milk of your choice

- 1 large scoop of whey or pea protein vanilla flavoured

- 1 large banana (peeled)

- 1 Pink Lady apple (finely chopped for blending)

- 1 tbsp minute oats

- 1/2 cup ice if you prefer a cold drink

Instructions

1. Soak minute oats in water for 10 minutes before blending

2. Blend water/milk with chia seeds, protein powder, banana, and chopped apple in a blender until all ingredients are smooth

3. Serve with a sprig of mint

Mango Prawn Poke Bowl

Preparation time

10 minutes

Ingredients

- 1 large avocado cut into chunks

- 1 mango cut into chunks

- 2 1/2 cups white basmati rice

- 6 tablespoons peeled shredded carrot

- 400 grams cooked prawns chopped into small bites (replace with 400 grams of Soyco® Thai tofu for vegans)

- 50 grams spinach leaves

- 1/2 cup finely chopped parsley

Dressing

- 1 teaspoon lemongrass pulp

- 1 teaspoon powdered garlic

- 60 ml extra virgin olive oil

- 50 ml fresh lime juice

- salt and pepper to taste

Instructions

1. For each bowl, arrange the ingredients white rice, mango chunks, avocado, shredded carrot, prawns (or tofu), baby spinach leaves, separately then sprinkle chopped parsley on top.

2. In a clean jar add the dressing ingredients and firmly close the lid and give them a good shake to blend the mixture, pour an even portion over the ingredients in each bowl.

Beetroot Carrot Salad

Preparation time

1 hour 10 minutes

Ingredients

- 3 golden beetroots (peeled) or 3 large carrots (skin left on) or mixture of both

- 500 grams haloumi (thickly sliced)

- 1 teaspoon fresh oregano leaves

- 100 ml maple syrup

- 50 ml fresh lemon juice

- 50 grams spinach leaves

- 200 grams hulled tahini

- 100 grams Chang's crispy noodles

- 2 tablespoons extra virgin olive oil

Instructions

1. Preheat the oven for 10 minutes at 180C.

2. Wrap the beetroot and/or carrots in foil and place in the oven for 40 minutes or until cooked through.

3. Put aside to cool then cut into wedges.

4. In a saucepan, heat olive oil to a medium heat and brown the haloumi on both sides.

5. Turn the heat down and add the maple syrup, lemon juice and oregano and stir through.

6. Place a tablespoon of hulled tahini on each serving plate and a few baby spinach leaves on top, then add the haloumi and the beetroot/carrot wedges.

7. Sprinkle with crispy noodles and top with left over juice.

Beetroot Tarte Tatin

Preparation time

53 minutes

Ingredients

- 8 small pre-cooked fresh beetroots thickly sliced

- 1 sheet thawed frozen puff pastry

- 8 basil leaves

- 50 grams crumbled feta cheese

- 1 tablespoon brown sugar

- 1 tablespoon balsamic vinegar

- 15 grams butter

Instructions

1. Preheat the oven to 200C fan forced

2. Grease a 24 cm pie tin.

3. Add butter, sugar, vinegar and beetroot to a heavy based fry pan and simmer and stir for approximately 15 mins until the liquid is thick.

4. Beetroots may crumble and the sauce caramelises. Let cool.

5. Place the beetroot pieces into the pie dish and top with pastry.

6. Bake for approximately 25 minutes until the pastry is golden and puffed.

7. When ready remove from oven and let cool for 10 minutes before turning out onto a serving plate.

8. Top the beetroot with basil leaves and crumbled feta.

Fresh Fricos

Preparation time

40 minutes

Ingredients

- 750 grams Coliban potatoes (washed and grated)

- 1 tablespoon finely chopped chives

- 1/2 teaspoon powdered garlic

- 50 mls Extra virgin olive oil

- 1/2 teaspoon dried rosemary

- 80 grams grated cheese (Montasio if you prefer a more Italian flavour)

- salt and pepper to taste

Instructions

1. Preheat the oven to 180C fan forced

2. In a large heavy bottomed saucepan add the olive oil and heat to medium, add the onion cook for a minute and add the potato.

3. Continuously toss the potato and onion, and season with salt and pepper.

4. Cook until the potato surfaces are golden and crispy.

5. Grease a 6-hole muffin tray, add the mixture until each hole is full, and press it down into the holes with the back of a spoon.

6. Bake for 20 minutes until the Fricos appear golden

7. Serve with some crispy steamed vegetables with a drizzle of olive oil salt and pepper to taste

Apple Blueberry Friands

Preparation time

45 minutes

Ingredients

- 50 grams almond meal

- 1/2 cup white plain flour

- 1/4 cup white self-raising flour

- 2 whole red apples (peeled, cooked and pureed)

- 1/2 cup blueberries (fresh or frozen)

- 5 egg whites

- 1/3 cup milk of your choice

- 3 tbsp stevia powder

- 1 tsp vanilla essence

- 1/4 cup grapeseed oil

Instructions

1. Lightly spray silicon friand moulds with oil of your choice, preheat the oven to 200C

2. In a large bowl mix all the flours and almond meal, stevia and vanilla essence until combined

3. Add milk of your choice and oil, apple and blueberries until evenly distributed.

4. In a separate bowl beat the egg whites until they form soft peaks and gently fold into the other mixture.

5. Spoon the mixture into the mould and turn heat down to 180C and bake for 20-30 minutes until the middle of the friand bounces back.

6. Let rest for 5 minutes before removing from mould tray and serve.

Roasted Apple and Veggies

Preparation time

1 hour 12 minutes

Ingredients

- 2 parsnips (peeled and sliced thickly length ways)

- 1 large carrot (peeled and sliced thickly length ways)

- 2 large red skinned potatoes (peeled and cut into chunks)

- 2 large red apples (cored and sliced into four)

- 4 sprigs of Thyme* (leaves separated from the twig)

- 4 tbsp extra virgin olive oil

- cracked salt and pepper to taste

Instructions

1. Heat oven to 180C for 20 minutes

2. Place all ingredients in a large bowl and coat with olive oil and ensure the vegetables are

coated with the oil and thyme leaves (or powder)

3. Place contents on baking paper in a baking tray and cook for 40-50 minutes until th

4. Enjoy with your favourite winter meals

Winter Apple Poke Bowl

Preparation time

54 minutes

Ingredients

- 1/2 butternut pumpkin (peeled and chopped)

- 1 red apple (finely sliced)

- 1 sachet precooked basmati rice (microwavable)

- 1/2 cup chopped chives

- 1/2 cup parsley and coriander (finely chopped)

- 200 grams haloumi (diced)

- Sprigs of parsley to decorate

- 2 tbsp extra virgin olive oil

- 2 tbsp lemon juice

- 1 tbsp honey

- 1 tsp grated ginger

Instructions

1. Heat an oven to 200C and place butternut pumpkin on baking paper and bake until golden approximately 30-40 minutes

2. Heat a non-stick pan to medium and add haloumi and cook until golden

3. When the pumpkin and haloumi are ready

4. Mix heated heated rice and all the other ingredients together in a bowl, mix through so all the ingredients are evenly distributed

5. Place the rice mix in the bowl and top with pumpkin and haloumi

6. Blend the dressing ingredients together and pour dressing over the top of the salad and garnish with parsley sprig

Miso Apple Soup

Preparation time

15 minutes

Ingredients

- 400 ml water

- 1/2 green apple (peeled, cored and grated)

- 100 grams pre cooked rice noodles

- 2 sachet single serve miso paste

- 1/4 cup chopped green chives

- 2 finely sliced mushrooms*

- 100 grams silken tofu crumbed

- 1 slice crispy roasted seaweed

Instructions

1. Rinse the rice noodles thoroughly in hot water and strain

2. Gently heat water to about 80 degrees

3. Add all ingredients except miso paste and stir for a minute or two until ingredients are warmed through

4. Add the two sachets of miso paste and blend through

5. Top with crushed seaweed flakes

Pancake Perfection

Preparation time

8 minutes

Ingredients

- 1/2 cup plain flour

- 3/4 cup milk of your choice

- 2 tablespoons oil (preferably olive oil)

- 1 cup of low fibre fruit – fresh (peeled and no pips or skin) or tinned (drained)

- pinch of salt

- maple syrup to drizzle

- cinnamon to decorate

Instructions

1. Add flour, crushed nuts pinch of salt and oil in a bowl and mix until completely smooth

2. Heat a greased shallow pan on medium

3. Gently pour a quarter of the mix into the pan and cook for 2-3 minutes then flip and cook on the other side

4. Repeat until all pancakes are made

5. Fold two pancakes into quarters arrange on each plate and add ½ cup of fruit on top and drizzle with maple syrup, sprinkle with cinnamon

Pesto Salmon

Preparation time

25 minutes

Ingredients

- 4 slices skin on salmon

- 4 1/2 slices of fresh lemon

- 1 sprig fresh parsley

- 120 grams pesto

- 200 grams snow peas (trimmed &deveined)

- 2 2 medium carrots (julienned)

- 2 packets white basmati microwavable rice

- Extra virgin olive oil

- salt and pepper to taste

Instructions

1. Heat the grill to medium.

2. Line a baking tray with foil and lightly baste the foil with olive oil.

3. Put the salmon, skin-side down, on the tray and add some pesto to each piece spreading it evenly across the top.

4. Lightly grill the salmon pieces for about 8 minutes for a pink inside, or longer depending on your preference.

5. Heat the rice as per the packet directions.

6. Lightly steam the carrots and snow peas and add them to the rice and toss through, add another teaspoon of pesto to flavour the grains, salt and pepper to taste.

7. Divide the rice into four bowls and place the salmon on top of each bowl.

8. Squeeze some fresh lemon on top of each piece of salmon and serve with slice of lemon and some parsley leaves.

Pasta Bake

Preparation time

55 minutes

Ingredients

- 500 grams peeled pumpkin or sweet potato cut into chunks

- 200 grams tinned asparagus cut into chunks

- 400 grams pasta

- 50 grams white bread broken up into crumbs

- 2 tablespoons oil (preferably olive oil)

- 400 mls vegetable or chicken stock

- 150 grams grated cheese

- 1 teaspoon mixed herbs

Instructions

1. Preheat the oven to 220C (fan forced)

2. Place the pumpkin/sweet potato in a baking dish and drizzle with one tablespoon of olive oil and roast until the vegetables soft and golden

3. At the same time boil the pasta until al dente and drain

4. In a bowl add breadcrumbs, stock, and the rest of the olive oil, mix until breadcrumbs dissolve then add asparagus, pumpkin, mixed herbs, add pasta and mix 100 grams of the cheese through

5. Place in a baking dish and heat through for 30 minutes finish off with the last 50 grams of cheese on top of the dish for 10 minutes until melted

6. Serve with salad or steamed greens

Cheesy Apple Toastie

Preparation time

13 minutes

Ingredients

- 1 slice Swiss cheese such as Edam, Gouda or Emmental

- 4 thin slices of red apple

- 2 slices white bread (or gluten free bread)

- olive oil spray

Instructions

1. Preheat the sandwich maker

2. Spray both sides of both piece of bread lightly

3. Make the sandwich by placing the apple slices on the bottom piece of bread and cheese on top

4. Add the top piece of bread

5. Close the sandwich maker and toast until golden

Apple Crisps

Preparation time

55 minutes

Ingredients

- 4 red skinned apples (peeled and cored)

- coconut oil spray

- cinnamon (optional)

Instructions

1. Preheat the oven to 140C fan forced

2. Slice the apples very thinly through the core to get really thin slices

3. Line a baking tin with baking paper and spray with coconut oil

4. Place the apple slices on the tray do not overlap, spray with coconut oil, if they overlap place extra in separate tray

5. Bake for 40 minutes until the slices are crispy (If you need two trays,   at 20minutes into baking swap bottom tray to top tray to ensure equal cooking)

6. Sprinkle with cinnamon

Serving suggestions

1. Float on top of a hot herbal tea

2. Crush and top salads

3. Place on top of chicken or pork dishes

4. Top a breakfast cereal with the crisps for an extra crunch

Fritter Fix

Preparation time

15 minutes

Ingredients

- 350 grams canned tuna or salmon (drained)

- 2 tablespoons oil (preferably olive oil)

- 50 grams tomato paste

- 400 grams cooked white rice (basmati if possible)

- 1/2 teaspoon paprika

- 1/2 cup minute oats (optional)

- 1/4 cup wholemeal flour

- 1 egg

Instructions

1. Heat the oven to 100C

2. Place rice in a large bowl add minute oats, fish, and paprika and mix thoroughly.

3. Make a well and add the beaten egg and tomato paste and blend until a soft mixture add white flour

4. Form eight fritters

5. Gently heat oil in a pan and add four fritters and cook until golden brown on both sides

6. Place in the oven to keep warm

7. Repeat and cook the last four

8. Serve with a crispy salad and a tablespoon of tomato sauce where possible

Egg Nests

Preparation time

20 minutes

Ingredients

- 6 free range eggs

- 6 slices white bread

- 1/4 cup chopped parsley or (1 tablespoon of dried parsley)

- extra virgin olive oil

- ground sea salt and pepper

Instructions

1. Preheat oven to 200C

2. Grease a muffin tray

3. Cut crusts off the bread and press one slice into each muffin mold

4. Place tray into the oven for 5 minutes until bread starts to crisp

5. Beat eggs add chopped/dried parsley

6. Pour eggs evenly into each of the molds and bake until the egg content is firm to the touch (5-10 minutes)

7. Add freshly ground sea salt and pepper to serve

Nutty Pudding

Preparation time

1 hour 20 minutes

Ingredients

- 200 grams tinned pear, peach or apple

- 25 grams crushed cashew nuts*

- 1 tablespoon vanilla extract

- vanilla pod (halved)

- 200 ml whole milk of your choice

- 1/2 teaspoon allspice mix

- 1/2 citrus fruit zest

- 75 grams spread of your choice

- 8 slices slightly stale white bread

- 3 free range eggs

- 2 tablespoons sugar or maple syrup or (1 tablespoon of stevia)

- 100 ml cream or coconut cream

Instructions

1. Heat the oven to 180C

2. Gently simmer milk in a small pan add vanilla extract and citrus zest and leave to cool

3. Thinly butter slices of bread on both sides and cut into quarters

4. Mash the fruit in a separate bowl

5. Lay the bread out in the base of the oven dish and add the layer of fruit and crushed nuts

6. Overlap the rest of the bread slices until all slices are used

7. Whip the eggs together with your sugar or sugar substitute add the milk, vanilla and citrus liquid and add cream, whip together until well blended, taste to ensure it is to your desired sweetness

8. Pour over the pudding and leave soak in to 20 minutes

9. Sprinkle the top with all spice

10. Place the oven dish into a roasting tin and fill the roasting tin with water to half way up the side of the pudding dish

11. Cook for 30-40 minutes until pudding is moist but firm

12. Let stand for 5 minutes and serve with vanilla ice cream or yoghurt

Sicilian Pizza

Preparation time

25 minutes

Ingredients

- 4 slices Tortilla bread (or similar)

- 190 grams canned tuna (drained)*

- 2 tablespoons oil (preferably olive oil)

- 90 grams pizza sauce

- 110 grams pitted olives

- 2 finely sliced mushrooms

- 1 cup grated cheese

- fresh or dried basil leaves

Instructions

1. Preheat the oven to 220C fan forced

2. Drain tuna and break into chunks

3. Top each 'pizza' base with pizza sauce, olives, mushrooms and tuna.

4. Bake for 10 minutes

5. Add cheese to each pizza and bake for a further 5 minutes to melt the cheese.

6. When cooked drizzle olive oil over and sprinkle with dried or fresh basil leaves

Zucchini Lasagne

Preparation time

1 hour

Ingredients

- 800 grams grated zucchini

- 1 teaspoon powdered onion

- 1 teaspoon powdered garlic

- 1 tablespoon chopped chives

- 1 tablespoon dried oregano

- 250 grams low-fat ricotta (or Tofutti*)

- 50 grams fat reduced shredded cheddar (or Sheese*)

- 350 ml passata

- 9 dried lasagne sheets (gluten free if needed*)

- extra virgin oil

- salt and pepper to taste

Instructions

1. Preheat the oven to 210C

2. Heat olive oil in a large fry pan and add onion and garlic powder, and zucchini, cook for 3 minutes

3. Turn the heat down and stir in ¾ tub of ricotta and 25 grams of reduced fat cheddar cheese (or vegan versions) add a little salt and pepper to taste – put aside

4. Boil lasagne sheets in water add a pinch of salt for about 5-6 minutes until just soft, but not fully cooked, drain and add some olive oil to the pasta to stop it sticking and to coat the layers

5. In a baking dish place a layer of lasagne sheet, then ricotta and zucchini mix, sprinkle each layer with oregano and chives, then a layer of tomato passata

6. Repeat layering until all lasagne and mixture is used

7. Add the rest of the ricotta to the top of the lasagne and sprinkle with cheddar cheese (or vegan version)

8. Turn the oven down to 180C

9. Bake the lasagne for 30 minutes until the pasta is soft and the top of the lasagne is golden

10. Serve with salad leaf salad

Pumpduken

Preparation time

1 hour 40 minutes

Ingredients

- 1 cup milk

- 2 kg peeled butternut pumpkin

- 1/3 cup smooth peanut butter

- 1 1/2 cup cooked basmati rice

- 2 teablespoons chopped chives

- 1 teaspoon dried garlic

- 100 grams crumbled feta

- 1 beaten egg

- 2 teaspon chopped rosemary leaves

- 1 Large *red capsicum halved and deseeded

- 1 long zucchini halved and deseeded (to make a well in each side)

- 1/2 cup carrot finely chopped

- String to tie the pumpduken

- Tomato passata with a dash of Worcestershire sauce to serve

- Extra virgin olive oil for basting

Instructions

1. Preheat the oven to 180C

2. Cut the peeled pumpkin in half and bake for 20 minutes until tender, take out of the oven

3. Scrape the middle out of each pumpkin half to make a well leaving a 2 cms thick outer wall of the pumpkin for the inner ingredients, set aside

4. In a heavy bottomed pan heat some olive oil, soften add dried garlic and chives stir through then add rosemary leaves

5. Mix rice, onion, garlic, fetta, and egg in a large bowl

6. Press the mixture down inside the pumpkin, leave a little of the mixture for packing around the inner vegetables

7. Press the capsicum halves, one in each side of the pumpkin and press down

8. Mix chopped carrot and smooth peanut butter together in a bowl

9. Place a zucchini half inside the capsicum and fill with chopped carrot and peanut butter mixture

10. Fill the remaining space between the capsicum and zucchini with the last of the rice mixture

11. Press everything down and gently place two halves of the pumpkin together and tie with string to keep together

12. Place on a baking tray and bake for 50-60 minutes until pumpkin is soft to touch

13. Gently remove the string and cut into slices and serve on with tomato salsa

Caprese Bocconcini Skewers

Preparation time

20 minutes

Ingredients

- 220 grams Bambini (or cherry) bocconcini

- Basil leaves

- 16 x 2cm cubes watermelon (no seeds)

- Balsamic glaze

- Wooden skewers

Instructions

1. Skewer melon ball first then a folded basil leaf then a bocconcini ball, followed by another folded basil leaf and a final melon ball

2. Lie skewers flat on a long dish and repeat until all ingredients are used

3. Drizzle a zig zag of balsamic glaze down the centre of the skewers and serve

Quick Creamy Prawn Pasta

Preparation time

20 minutes

Ingredients

- 350 grams dry wholemeal penne pasta

- 2 tablespoon unsalted butter

- 1/2 cup chicken stock

- 1/2 cup chives (finely minced)

- 500 grams shelled deveined raw prawns

- 100 grams plain Greek yoghurt

- 1 cup baby spinach

- 1 lemon zest

- Salt and pepper to taste

Instructions

1. Cook pasta and drain in a heavy bottomed pot

2. In a deep fry pan melt butter and add chives and lightly braise until they are soft

3. Add chicken stock and simmer for 5 minutes to reduce volume

4. Add prawns, lemon zest and toss through the onion until the prawns are cooked on a low heat

5. Add yoghurt a little salt and pepper to the drained pasta and warm on a low heat

6. Toss in prawn mix and spinach and stir through until well mixed

7. Serve while warm

Yoco Dessert

Preparation time

4 hours 10 minutes

Ingredients

- 700 grams greek yoghurt

- 1 teaspoon vanilla essence

- 200 ml low-fat buttermilk

- 2 tablespoon pure honey

- 2 tablespoon cornflakes

- grated dark chocolate

Instructions

1. Whisk yoghurt, honey, buttermilk and vanilla essence together

2. Place in a freezer safe container and freeze for 3-4 hours

3. If the dessert is too hard to serve leave out for 5-10 minutes to soften and scoop into dishes

4. Top with shaved chocolate and crunchy cornflakes

Notato chips

Preparation time

1 hour 17 minutes

Ingredients

- 7 peeled medium radishes

- 1/2 teaspoon garlic powder

- 1/2 teaspoon cumin

- spray olive oil

- 1 pinch Himalayan salt

- 1 pinch fresh black pepper

Instructions

1. Pre heat the oven to 220C

2. Finely slice the peeled radishes into thin slivers

3. Place them in a bowl add garlic powder, salt, cumin and black pepper and spray with olive oil Mix thoroughly until the radishes are coated

4. Place on an oven tray with no overlapping areas so they can crisp easily

5. Bake for about an hour until they are crisp and golden

6. Cool and serve